Lose The Fat Spell

And Feel Great

By
BenedikteEva

DEDICATION

To Garfield the cat

ACKNOWLEDGMENTS

I want to acknowledge the World Health Organization (WHO) and
http://www.worldometers.info/weight-loss/ for providing me with
useful facts and numbers about overweight and obesity

1 PROLOGUE

The wicked witch

Once upon a time an extremely powerful witch cast a spell on me. This powerful witch was me.
The spell the wicked witch cast was this:

"You're fat, and you need to lose some weight"

And I looked at myself in the mirror and thought: "yes, I am fat and I need to lose some weight"

At that time I was 13. Before that I also thought of myself as not thin, but it was not something I thought much about. My parents were not exactly slim, and my mother's parents were fat people and had been as long as I can remember. They were wonderful people so I just loved them and enjoyed their company, as any grandchild should enjoy their grandparents, without having any prejudices about their degree of fatness.

My mother went to the doctor with me at some point. Not because I was sick or she was, just for a checkup. She herself wanted to talk about a diet for herself. Then suddenly she says to the doctor that she thinks that I could need to lose some weight too and asks if he could suggest a diet for me.

I felt I was in the twilight zone. Haven't seen this coming at all. Here I ran around knowing that I wasn't thin but didn't care much about it and then suddenly it was something that would change my life. I should go on a diet, eat more vegetables and less candy. I didn't quite know the implications of this ordeal but I felt both angry and scared.

My grandparents had a summerhouse where we went for a couple of weeks every summer. When my grandparents tucked me and my brothers in at night, my grandfather would tell us a story and my grandmother would come and give us a chocolate box filled with different kinds of candy, and we would eat that while my grandpa told the story. I loved it, and there my evenings were wonderful, safe and funny. Even now when I eat some candy I can get that feeling of warmth, safety and happiness.

That was going to be taken away from me.

I don't think my mother knew what I was experiencing during this doctors' appointment, and I am pretty sure that she meant me only well, but that day it felt like my world was falling apart. It was that day, I went home, looked myself in the mirror and thought: "yes I am fat and I need to lose some weight"

And what I created there has been the truth ever since, except when I was sixteen and just had had the flu, and lost a couple of kilos, and there were no fat left on my waistline. The other time was period of time that started 1 year after my son was born where I weighed 108 kg.

Breaking the fat spell the first time

At that point in life I had been on a lot of different diets since I was 13 and I was now 29 years old, and in that period of time I had more than doubled my weight. Some of it came from growing in height, bosom and hips which is quite normal when you are between 13 and 20. The rest of it was just excess fat.

Then I had the following realization: "Okay I have been on diets for 16 years now and I have gained more than 50 kg's in that period of time, maybe it is time to stop dieting, because it clearly doesn't work".

So I stopped being on a diet, started to walk a lot, made some minor changes to my daily eating like changing the butter type to one with less calories and the bread I was eating to something with more fibers, but continued like I had always eaten and that was enough and I lost 25 kg's in 3 years.

In about ten years I weighed between 80-85 kg's and I am 175 cm tall so, well I wasn't slim or anything but I could run, play soccer with my son and felt I was in better shape than ever and was definitely not dieting.

Then I turned 40, stopped smoking, met my boyfriend, started drinking wine in the weekends (good food, good wine), gained 2 kg, looked at myself in the mirror and thought: 'yes, I am fat, and need to lose some weight', and gained an additional 25 kg over the next 2 years.

At this point I am 42 and weigh 110 kg, and am under my fat spell once more.

And a lot of other people in the world might be under a similar spell. I will give you some facts I found on the internet on obesity on the following page.

Fact from WHO (World Health Organization)'s homepage:

> **"More than 1.4 billion adults were overweight in 2008, and more than half a billion obese**
>
> *In 2008, more than 1.4 billion adults were overweight and more than half a billion were obese. At least 2.8 million people each year die as a result of being overweight or obese. The prevalence of obesity has nearly doubled between 1980 and 2008. Once associated with high-income countries, obesity is now also prevalent in low- and middle-income countries".*
>
> From: http://www.who.int/features/factfiles/obesity/en/

In Denmark it is recently discovered that more than 50 % of the Danish population is overweight.

> *"Once associated with high-income countries, obesity is now also prevalent in low- and middle-income countries".*
>
> *http://www.who.int/features/factfiles/obesity/en/*

From 1980 and until now the diet-industry has grown large, and people along with it. Maybe it is time to think differently about body weight issues.

On this page http://www.worldometers.info/weight-loss/ it is visualized that almost every second one person is getting a BMI on more than 25.

And here is a quote from the same page:

Spending on weight-loss programs and products in the USA

*According to the U. S. Food and Drug Administration (FDA)
Americans spent an estimated **$30 billion a year in 1992** on all types
of diet programs and products, including diet foods and drinks.*

*Market data, a market research firm that has tracked diet products
and programs since 1989 releases its findings in its biennial study:
"The U.S. Weight Loss & Diet Control Market." which in its **2007**
study estimates the size of the U.S. weight loss market at **$55
billion**. It is now estimated to have reached **over $60 Billion**.*

This book is not an attack on the diet industry or on people who try
to make a living out of helping people lose weight. But since the
facts are like they are, maybe people working in the diet industry
might take the ideas in this book into consideration, when making
their next diet, remedy or weight loss program.

---

*"Overweight and obesity are defined as abnormal or excessive fat
accumulation that presents a risk to health. A crude population
measure of obesity is the body mass index (BMI), a person's weight
(in kilograms) divided by the square of his or her height (in meters).
A person with a BMI of 30 or more is generally considered obese. A
person with a BMI equal to or more than 25 is considered
overweight".*

From WHO's homepage: http://www.who.int/topics/obesity/en/index.html

---

If you do a lot of exercise and have great muscle mass then BMI can
be misleading.

2 THE FAT SPELL

The purpose of this book is to break my own fat spell and help others break theirs, and thereby free the people and create joy and vitality.

Spells are beliefs in the form of a sentence of words, which are repeated over and over again in our mind or in our surroundings.

A spell serves as part of a visualization. It sets the unconscious in motion to create exactly the situation, event or item it describes, at least in our minds. The visualization comes from the pictures, emotions and/ or sounds you think of when hearing the words.

Beliefs are that which shape our experience of life, and points the direction of our life and also create the limitations to what we can or cannot do.

Habits

When we do things in our lives that we have done repeatedly every day, we often do it automatically. We don't need to think about it. As an example walking, dressing, eating, drinking, brushing our teeth etc. This is a good thing because if we had to relearn as an example walking every morning things could get really difficult.

The same goes for eating. This is an unconscious process, a habit, most of the time, and what we eat, and how we eat is decided partly from our automatic behaviors, and partly on what is available to us. Our automated behavior comes from how we believe the world is and we act according to these beliefs.

Body image

The body image you hold in your can be very different from what other people see. If you have an eating disorder where your BMI gets lower than 20, then you might still say: 'I am fat and need to lose weight', which in that case you don't. In that case the body image in your mind and your factual body, don't have much in common.

This is not just people with an eating disorder who don't see their real body. In a TV-show I watched about learning how to dress so you looked the best, they line up a bunch of women of different sizes in their underwear. Then one woman who wants to do something about her style must choose what size waistline and but matches hers. It is very common that women think they are two sizes bigger than they really are.

Body image is something that rarely fits the actual body.

If we then look at the body image from the outside, what other people see, this is a different story as well. Men often don't see the extra kilos on women stomachs, but only bosoms, buts and hips and a lot of guys enjoy a good handful of those parts. Girls might notice if a guy is obese, especially when there is a risk of him getting a heart attack during intercourse, but a few extra can be quite sexy.

Then there is the other end of weight issues where you end up being obese with a BMI of more than 35. I do not know what kind of body image people have when they get there, but I know from myself with a BMI on 35,9 that I don't think of myself as obese. Yeah I am overweight but I am not obese. In my mind I have the same size I had when I was 17 and I am often chocked when I accidentally catch a glimpse of my reflection in a shop window.

From the front I look okay, but from the side I can see that I am actually a big mama.

I don't believe I have an eating disorder, but know I am under the fat spell big time.

The fat spell and its variations

The fat spell can have a lot of variations but basically looks like this:

"I am X and I Y to lose weight"

Where the X stands for overweight, fat or obese (or similar) and the Y stands for should, ought to, want to, have to, need to or I die if I don't (or similar).

I am	X	And I	Y	Lose weight
			Ought to	
	overweight		Want to	
I am	fat	And I	Have to	lose weight
	Obese		Should	
	?(fill in)		Need to	
			die if I don't	
			? (fill in)	

The fat spell is not necessarily related to anything in the body, only to the image we have of our own body in our mind and to our definition of fat. If our body image is fat, and we believe that having a fat body is unhealthy, ugly, unlovable, unattractive or socially unacceptable then we often believe weight loss will be necessary to be healthy, socially accepted, loved and good looking.

Explanatory beliefs

There are often other beliefs attached to the fat spell; beliefs that serve as reason to why you should or have/want/need/ought to lose some weight.

So here is the revised formula:

I am X and I Y to lose weight because Z

I am X and I Y to lose weight because	Z
I am X and I Y to lose weight because	*It is unhealthy to be fat.* *fat is ugly* *overweight causes disease* *my partner will leave me if I'm fat* *I want to be a model, and models must be thin* *someone tells me to* *? (fill in)*

Often the fat spell is accompanied by a reason why we are not successful about losing the extra weight:

I'm X and I Y lose weight, because Z, but I can't because V

V stands for: I have no will power/ can't resist, have the backbone of a jellyfish and similar

I am X and I Y to lose weight because Z, and I can't lose weight because	V
	I have the backbone of a jellyfish
	Can't resist
	Have no will power
I am X and I Y to lose weight because Z, and I can't lose weight because	my partner or parent makes to good food
	I am not motivated
	I have no discipline
	I can't exercise
	I am addicted to food
	Nothing works
	? (fill in)

Well you can come up with a number of different reasons to why you should lose weight and why you can't. But basically if you are under the fat spell, there is either something wrong with overweight and/or you feel there is something wrong with you.

You might also have the belief that: "I'm fat and I'm proud of it/feel great/ and so what". Or you might not believe you're fat at all. Congratulations you don't have the fat spell.

You might have other spells and you can work with them in the same way, so please read on.

A day under the fat spell

If we believe ourselves to be fat and needing to lose weight, this will be the concept of reality we eat ourselves in to.

It works in my life as this. My meals are healthy, but as soon I don't pay attention I almost automatically puts something like candy in my head, or put a little extra on my plate for dinner, and then think if I notice what I'm doing: "just this once can't hurt" but if I do that every day the result is that I stay in the reality of fatness.

So when under the fat spell, a lot of the things you do and the thoughts you think and even your mood will be determined by the spell.

Here is an example of a day under the fat spell from my life:

I wake up in the morning, swing my legs out of bed, and look at my protruding belly, and think: I should really lose some weight. Then I put on my lenses, step on the scale, and if I lost a little weight I think: it is probably not permanent, or if it is the same as the day before I think: at least I haven't gained weight or if I have gained weight I think: oh no I am getting fatter I should be more careful about what I eat, and my mood drops a bit.

Then I put some clothes and look in the mirror and whether I'm in a good, neutral or bad mood I think I am fat and need to lose weight.

Then I have breakfast. A couple of wholegrain buns with a thin layer of butter and thin slices of cheese or ham or a thin layer of jam on top, with some coffee and juice, and sometimes fruit.

Lot of people under the fat spell would skip that meal, but since I have the belief that not eating will lower your metabolism I figure that a healthy breakfast is important. So breakfast is one of the things I will think about because I am fat and need to lose some weight that will keep the kilos of my hips.

After breakfast I usually walk for an hour, to clear my mind and because I am fat and need to lose weight. It is a good thing to get some fresh air before writing for hours but it is also partly determined by the fat spell.

It is the time that comes after breakfast and the walk where my actions reinforce the fat spell.

When I write I have a tendency to make a lot of displacement activity and that often involves eating. Every time I do a displacement activity involving food (except when it is fruit or similar) then I think I shouldn't do this, cause I am fat and I need to lose weight. With the first act of procrastination I think: one little piece of chocolate can't hurt, but if you make a lot of these displacement activities a day, then you end up being fat and needing to lose weight, at least that is what I think every time I have done this automatic behavior.

Then I eat lunch. And again I eat something that is not a problem, dark bread with some low fat meat on it, and a tomato or avocado, perfectly all right, and it is the right thing to do if you are fat and need to lose weight. But after lunch I feel a little tired and look down at my protruding stomach and think: I'm fat and need to lose weight".

This continues all day, and I eat a healthy meal in the evening (most of the time) and when I automatically put that little extra on my plate and accidently notice it I think: "this can't hurt just this once". And after the meal when I sit there feeling completely stuffed I think: "I am fat and need to lose weight" and then it time for desert and bed.

So the days and the weeks and the months and the years continue under that spell and I'm getting fatter and really need to lose some weight.

Of cause I do not think this line all the time, because I also have a lot of other things I do and think about, like writing books, singing, painting, being with my boyfriend, son and family, laughing and enjoying life. But the spell is there, playing its song over and over again, sometimes loud and sometimes low but still there. In just one day I might think a hundred times: "I am fat and want to/ should/ have to/ need to lose weight", and every time my spirit drops a bit, because I feel I'm not good enough, that there is something wrong with me, that I am not beautiful, sexy or healthy, etc.

But it is just a spell. When I was 17 I weighed 2 kilos more than my ideal weight which was the weight I have with a BMI on 22. And I also thought then: I am fat and I should lose weight.

The fat spell is not necessarily a question about you weight or how you look or how healthy you are, it is just a spell. In my case the spell became reality in the sense that I have gained a lot of weight since it was cast.

And why would I want to break it? Maybe I will lose some weight (and I am fat and need to lose some weight) or maybe I never will.

Just imagine this for a moment. If you are under the fat spell, there might be the risk that the weight you are carrying around now will be a part of you for the rest of your life. Imagine that your excess fat will stay there no matter what you do. Like a faithful dog that keeps following you around.

Can you accept and live with that situation?

The first time I broke the fat spell that was exactly what I did, accepted the situation as it was. I thought that since I have had this fat for so long and there has become more of it, and it is not likely to disappear tomorrow or any time soon, then I must learn to live with it. So I accepted my body image and me as was then and focused on getting in shape and enjoying life anyway.

Instead of looking at my fat I started to look at my intelligence, my great sense of humor and my smile, and thought: "wow I am pretty amazing". This was a new spell and after a couple of years I was in fair shape I could both run and play football, and I lost 25 kg in a few years.

4 REMEDIES AND DIETS

Another quote from WHO (World Health Organization)

"For an individual, obesity is usually the result of an imbalance between calories consumed and calories expended

An increased consumption of highly calorific foods, without an equal increase in physical activity, leads to an unhealthy increase in weight. Decreased levels of physical activity will also result in an energy imbalance and lead to weight gain"

http://www.who.int/features/factfiles/obesity/facts/en/index4.html

When you are under the fat spell, you might consider going on a diet or take some pills that should lessen the problem. And you probably want most of the fat gone in as little time as possible.

But it rarely works this way. I am not saying that diets and remedies don't help you lose weight because they do if you follow them.

What diets and remedies don't do is helping you to stay slim if you after the diet return to a way of living where you consume more calories than you use.

Spells of food

Another problem with diets is that there are a lot of different studies of the effects of various foods, which shows different things. These studies become beliefs or rather spells that flows through the air, making the act of eating something we think about all the time:

I shouldn't eat bananas because there is sugar in it and sugar makes you fatter. Or you should eat wholegrain and vegetables all the time to lose weight. Don't eat too much meat, because there are a lot of calories in it, eat only meat and eggs to build muscles. Carbohydrates are good, but not in the form of sugar, carbohydrates is fattening, fat is fattening, and fat is bad for you. You have to get some fat or your digestion stops. Eat lots of protein, stay away from meat. You must only eat one type of fat not another, stay away from sugar, sugar is dangerous for your weight, drink tons of water, don't drink wine, drink a glass of white wine to every meal that will heighten your metabolism, take this pill, make this exercise eat this eat that. Don't eat this and don't eat that, do this don't do that and so on.

Or here is a new pill mixture or program that will help you lose the extra kilos, and it is all scientifically proved. And just look at the before - after pictures. You want that right? (And the deadly side effects just happen to 10 % so don't worry (that was sarcasm)).

And all of that is scientifically proved whether or not they tell you completely opposite things. I get so stressed that I get an instant craving for chocolate, candy and cookies and lots of it, and then I can think I am fat and need to lose weight, and get depressed because I have absolutely no willpower and the backbone of a jellyfish and then I eat some more chocolate.

If you are under the fat spell you might focus a lot about your calorie intake, instead of enjoying the food.

Exercise could be measured by its fun value or the opportunity to hang out with other people, but instead the focus is on how many calories can be lost.

If we eat fewer calories than we use, in time we will lose weight. It is not a matter of the right diet; just use more than you eat. It is not so important whether you will do that by exercise more or eating less or both.

Then you can do this in a healthy way or in an unhealthy way, where you get proper nutrition or not or getting exercise or not.

With every kilo you lose you must remember that you also get less weight to carry around. And less weight takes fewer calories to lift and carry. So if you have regulated you daily calorie burning balance you might want to adjust that sometimes.

My point is that the principle of losing weight is easy and it really should be natural for us to adjust our bodies, to an adequate performance.

There is no right diet for the fat spell, and it will be there no matter how much weight you lose or gain or how you lose or gain it, unless of cause you lose the spell.

Another thing about diets

One assumption in any diet is that women should have no more than 2000 calories a day and men no more than 2500 on average. Note that IN AVERAGE A DAY. But sometimes we do lots of hard work and this takes more energy, and sometimes we do close to nothing, and we need less calories. We can't base our diets on an overall average. Each of us is individuals with unique bodies, lives, stories and metabolism. And days are different from each other (hopefully). To know when you have had enough to eat, is something that should be natural, but for some reason no longer is for a large part of the worlds' population. (And when I say large I mean it in the big sense). So we might want to start listen to our bodies, to feel that we had enough to eat.

5 WHY DO WE WANT TO LOSE WEIGHT?

A spell has certain results. As an example: having the fat spell results in having the idea that you are fat and want, need, have, ought to or should lose weight, no matter how much the actual weight is.

It controls some of your actions; your conscious choices and habitual choices. When you choose to eat healthy and low calorie then there will come a counteraction when you are not thinking about it to maintain the situation of the spell.

It also serves as a visualization that causes the situation to be true, whether it is only in the mind of the spell infected or in the actual body.

So if you are fat and need to lose weight then it is a very bad idea to visualize a picture of yourself as being fat, it is then most lightly to happen; at least your own version of fat.

Some people need severe obesity to consolidate the spell, while others let only a few extra kilos determine that they are fat and need to lose weight. Some again only needs to be able to grab a bit of skin to think they are fat and need to lose weight.

Obesity and overweight is about the weight in the sense that it puts a lot of strain on the body.

The fat spell is only in the mind, but can worsen the condition of overweight and obesity, and make it very difficult to do anything about it because the spell programs what you eat and how you eat, which is for the most part an automatic process and therefore affected by spells.

Making a wish

In chapter 2 I defined the fat spell and following examples on what would follow the line:

'I am X and I Y to lose weight because Z, but I can't because V'

If you want to make a spell and visualization for what you want rather than what you don't want then it might serve you well to actually figure out what you want.

If we look at the spell where there is some reason or a threat to why you should lose weight when you are fat then you can just add a wish afterwards. This is not a counter spell yet but your mind will begin a journey with another focus. A focus on what you want will change your direction.

'I am X and I Y to lose weight because Z, and I would really want W'

Where W stands for what you wish for. What you want.

As an example:

"I'm fat and want to lose weight because fat is ugly and I really want to be beautiful".

Here is the underlying wish to be beautiful. Or...

Now it is easy to think that we all want to beautiful, rich and so on, but for some beauty is not that important but they think that in order to be socially accepted or loved or whatever, their looks must meet certain standards. So the true wishes here is to be loved or socially accepted or whatever.

For me being beautiful is something I am sometimes, whether fat or thin, in both cases I can be beautiful or ugly. It depends mostly on my emotional state that day, and emotional states can be changed in an instant if you know how.

My personal fat spell with a number one reason goes like this:

"I'm fat and need to lose weight, because it is unhealthy being fat".

I am simply concerned about my health. It is not very important for me to be socially accepted, since I am an introvert person who rather wants to do a lot of stuff by myself instead of surrounding myself with a lot of people.

But it is important for me to be healthy. Not just to avoid pain and ailments, but to feel free, strong and full of joy and vitality, and live long and prosper.

The feeling of joy when running as fast as you can, the thrill of dancing wildly for a long time, and be able to live well passed a hundred, cause I really love life. This is my true wish, and this is what I want to visualize and eventually have instead of the fat spell.

To start me in a new direction my revised fat spell would be:

"I am fat and I want to lose weight because fat is unhealthy and I really want to feel free, strong and full of joy and vitality and live long and prosper"

Others might have the fat spell in other forms like:

I'm fat and I ought to lose weight, because fat is ugly, and when I'm are ugly nobody will love me"

So they really want to be loved. In that case you can make an efficient love spell. Love spells are not something you cast upon somebody else to make them love you. A love spell is something you cast on yourself to make you open for love. Fat is not a reason to why people can't love you, but your internal marketing department might be doing a poor job making you lovable to anybody especially yourself.

The revised spell could be:

"I am fat and I want to lose fat because fat is ugly, and when I'm are ugly nobody will love me, and I really want to be loved"

If love is what you want, then stop using fat as an excuse for not having love, and start giving your internal marketing department some new instructions; a new spell to run.

Like: I am such a wonderful person and so are you.

Spells doesn't have to be logical. They are just like background music playing out our beliefs. Our actions are determined by what we believe.

So play another song. A song about love, and health, beauty and joy and all the other stuff you want in your life, that is not measureable by a scale.

After you have found the wish in the fat spell then cross out the fat spell and let the wish stand on its own:

"~~I am fat and I want to lose weight because fat is unhealthy and~~ I really want to feel free, strong and full of joy and vitality and live long and prosper"

This is a powerful wish, and my wish is my command.

6 THE TREACHUROUS FAT SPELL

The Fat spell is treacherous. First it claims that it is a part of our being (I am X). Then it makes sure that we can't get rid of it by making itself fulfill itself by controlling our habitual acts like eating and choosing food and exercise when we are not aware of it. Then it makes us believe that there is something wrong with us because we are not losing the weight (but I can't lose weight because Z).

But remember this: My fat spell was once cast by me and you fat spell was first cast by you. We might have heard it from others: parents, friends or the media, but it is ours, and it is our own responsibility to try to create the life we want for ourselves.

It might be interesting if we started to look at weight as a part of our circumstances rather than a personal quality. And a part that is ours and which we can change.

The mix-up of the Fat Spell

In the last chapter I claimed that underneath the Z part; the 'because', lies something we want to get out of losing weight; the big W, a desire of ours. It can be love, health, beauty, social acceptance or a partner, a career or whatever we can think of.

But losing the weight won't ensure any of it, and the fulfillment of these desires might happen even if we don't lose weight.

It is like cleaning the floors and then expecting this act will get the dishes done. It's not going to happen, if you want the dishes done you must do the dishes, and if you want the floor clean you must clean the floor.

Weight loss is no guarantee for finding a partner, experience love, be socially accepted, being beautiful, having a great health or anything. In cases where the weight is followed by a lot of other health issues losing weight can minimize the health problems, but it is no guarantee.

It might help some people feel more confident and thereby help them get love and partners and jobs, but that is because of the increase in self-confidence not the weight loss.

And love, jobs, social acceptance and better health can happen anyway, no matter how your current weight situation is.

But we might have a tendency to hold back on the actions that can give us what we wish for, if our own requirements for what will cause the wishes to happen are not met: in this case if we believe we are fat and should lose some weight.

The weight spell sounds like it is a quality about you. "I am Fat" but the truth is that the 'I' in question is that particular 'I', no matter what weight it is carrying around. So the amount of fat on your body is just a circumstance and you can change that.

It takes time to do the dishes. If you have had a great dinner with your whole extended family it takes longer than it does if you have had a piece of toast for breakfast.

And losing the excess fat can be compared with the act of cleaning; in this case cleaning the body for the excess weight you carry around. And I am pretty sure that you do not have to think much about it when doing the dishes or cleaning to floor.

Or imagine that you have a plant on you table. It starts out as an ordinary sized plant and you nurture it. Now imagine that it grows 1 inch a day. Soon you will have to trim it or it will be all over the house in no time. Same goes for fat. You can have the amount of fat needed by the body or you can let it grow all over your body. But at some point you might feel that you do not have so much room left. Maybe it is time to trim the plants and do the dishes. And please take your time and do it lovingly.

7 THE GREAT SPELL

In the two previous chapters have tried to figure out what I really want, and now I can make a new spell to fulfill that wish.

With regards to the actual fat, then remember that your body and mind is actually capable self regulating over time if you let it, honestly eat a little less, exercise more. Give your mind new instructions like:

 "My body and mind work together in harmony creating joy, health, beauty and vitality".

Or

"I create health, beauty, love and vitality for myself and I enjoy life fully"

You can probably come up with other spells and affirmation that will work for your specific wishes, just remember two things.

1. Only say what you want, what you work towards, not what you don't want and want to move away from.

2. Don't make identity statements like "I am X "because you are just you not any kind of X. But you are able to create X.

The new spells you create are magic. And it works even better if you say it as a ritual. Where before you thought 'I am X and Y to lose weight" then think: "I create health, beauty, love and vitality for myself and I enjoy life fully" or "my body and mind works together in harmony creating joy, health, beauty and vitality" or whatever great spell you created.

Run it over in your mind before every meal, I know I will, and allow it to work, to be a habit and see what happens. You can make it a ringtone on your phone as a reminder. Or write it on your fridge or on your plates.

Make a painting of it, create a song or a dance of it can also help you put the new spell to work.

And then throw out the scale or at least put it away for a year and see what happens.

8. CONCLUSION

If the diet industry has grown in size and the number of overweight people is increasing every second, then the human race is handling the issue of overweight in a non efficient manner.

Overweight is an imbalance over time where we get more energy in than we use. The extra energy stays in the body as fat.

If we just use a little more energy than we get in over a period of time we will eventually correct the imbalance.

If our natural energy balance is disturbed by a spell (a belief we consolidate by repeating it and acting to fulfill) then we can start changing the spell and make a new one that works in our best interest.

Losing the fat spell might not cause weight loss, but keeping the fat spell without making new practices and thoughts of eating and exercise won't cause weight loss either.

So if you are weighed down psychologically by the fat spell, please lose that and create a better spell or affirmation that gives you a feeling of power and joy.

You might still want to deal with an energy imbalance, just remember that overweight is just a circumstance you can change, not something you are. Only you can change that circumstance.

Give yourself the time to change it. You might have lived with that circumstance for a long time, and it is not going away tomorrow.

Say your new spells before every meal or use mine if you like:

"My body and mind work together in harmony creating joy, health, beauty and vitality".

Or

"I create health, beauty, love and vitality for myself and I enjoy life fully"

I know i will

Love BenedikteEva

OTHER BOOKS BY BENEDIKTEEVA

Life of a Magician – Magical contact lenses 1

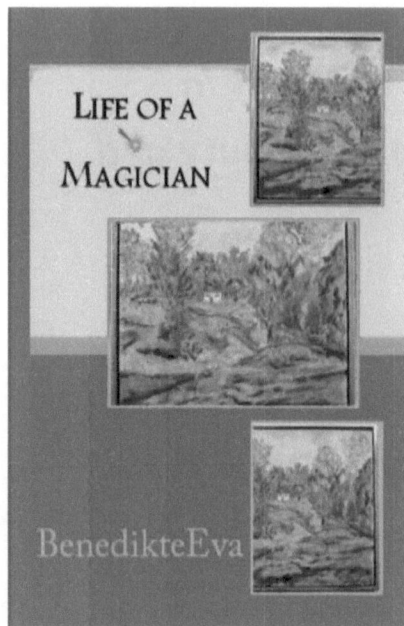

Imagine that you put on a pair of colored contact lenses. When you look at the world it then seem to be colored in the color of the lenses. After a while you get used to see the world like this and you do not notice the color anymore. Our beliefs about ourselves and the world are metaphorical equivalent to the color of the lenses, we are so used to, how the world looks, through our beliefs that we rarely stop to wonder how the world really is or if it could be different.

This book offers another set of metaphorical contact lenses that gives an opportunity to work with our life and experience, thought and feelings in a magical way.

Paperback 15 $: https://www.createspace.com/4143520

As PDF 7 $ (approximately at Saxo.dk)

For Kindle 8, 75 $

Book of Magic in Practice - Magical Contact Lenses 2

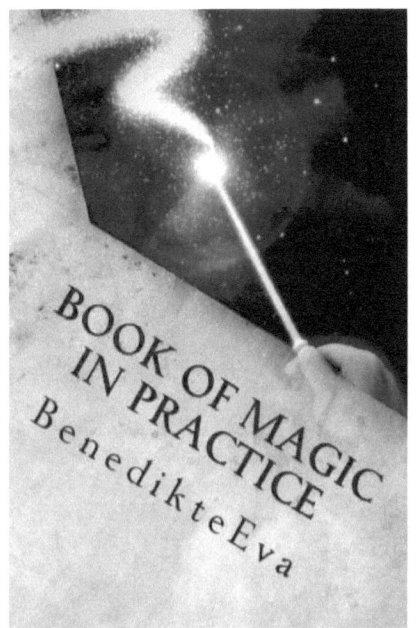

Book of Magic in Practice is the second book in the series With Magical Contact Lenses. The book describes how to use the filter of beliefs I call: 'Magical Contact Lenses' to create a living experience of the reader's own choice.

This book will take the reader through many kinds of magic and stages of reality, where magic action can happen.

The purposes of the book is to inspire vibrant, harmonic growth, expand human consciousness and do it in a way that leaves the reader free to create bubbly joy, love beyond imagination, flowing abundance or whatever overall state the reader wants to experience.

Paperback 17 $: https://www.createspace.com/4143529

As PDF   8, 75 $ (approximately at Saxo.dk)

For Kindle 8, 75$

ABOUT THE AUTHOR

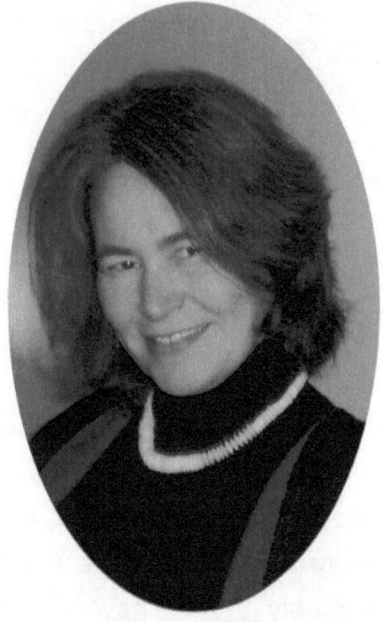

Magician, musician and artist with a skewed view of the world a love of jazz and a quiet nature loving mind.

www.ingramcontent.com/pod-product-compliance
Lightning Source LLC
Chambersburg PA
CBHW030549290526
45786CB00004B/1940